CHEWS
TO BE
Healthy

CHEWS TO BE *Healthy*

The Working Mom's Interactive
Guide for Disease and *Weight Control*

LAFARRA YOUNG, MD

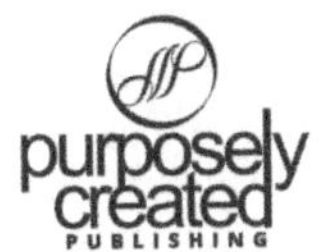

purposely
created
PUBLISHING

CHEWS TO BE HEALTHY

Published by Purposely Created Publishing Group™

Copyright © 2019 LaFarra Young

All rights reserved.

No part of this book may be reproduced, distributed or transmitted in any form by any means, graphic, electronic, or mechanical, including photocopy, recording, taping, or by any information storage or retrieval system, without permission in writing from the publisher, except in the case of reprints in the context of reviews, quotes, or references.

Printed in the United States of America

ISBN: 978-1-64484-055-9

DEDICATION

This book is dedicated to my parents and my three children. From the moment I met all of you, I started to become the person I am today. Mom and Dad, you taught me to respect and challenge myself even though I didn't learn for decades what that really meant. You believed in me even when I didn't believe in myself, and you challenged me to be grateful no matter what I was going through. Josh, Ben, and Lory, you taught me how to prioritize. I loved you from the day you became more than a thought. Even though I know you don't feel like it, you are truly my mini partners. The unconditional love that I am able to share with all of you makes me stronger and inspires me to be better. Living with an autoimmune disease has been so much easier because I have you all as a source of stability and love.

I am also grateful to my coach Dr. Drai who encouraged me to keep going because he believed in me, even though sometimes I didn't understand his "why" for pushing me. I am also grateful for Dr. Samm, my naturopathic doctor and my friend, for keeping me focused and helping me to heal. I get asked questions from individuals, often women, with similar issues to me about how to take care of themselves and their families. What diet and foods should they eat in order to be healthy or to feel better with certain diseases? As a health coach, I am blessed to aide clients no longer satisfied with just treating their symptoms but getting to the underlying cause and eliminating it through both diet (inner foods) and the outside environment (outer foods) influencing their bodies.

God has smiled on me, and it is with much humility that I express the ultimate gratitude for allowing me to become healthier and to overcome adversities I face daily. Thank You for your unwavering patience with me.

TABLE OF CONTENTS

FOREWORD

Dr. LaFarra has laid out a thorough explanation of what I have for years considered the root cause of many of our illnesses—inflammation. She has brilliantly explained this curse and shown us how it is linked as the cause or side effect of many common and not so common illnesses such high blood pressure and diabetes, or autoimmune conditions such as lupus and sarcoidosis.

I love how she takes her time to explain what these illnesses are and how they affect us.

As a board-certified pathologist and certified health coach, she has a unique perspective on health in general. Coupled with her ownership in a Cajun restaurant and love for food, she is overqualified to deliver this message of how you truly can use food as your medicine if you are willing to do the work.

She is painfully transparent in this book about her struggles with her own autoimmune issues and how she had to fight with her own demons to gain control of her diet and ultimately her health. She shares her journey of how she did this and now does this with her own clients.

It is said that you must be a student before you can be a teacher. She can speak on this topic because she has mastered it through trial and error, research, being the student (naturopathic patient), and finally receiving her certification to coach others.

Lastly, she gives amazing advice on how to practically and easily conquer the beast that we call inflammation using what she calls primary and secondary foods.

It is my sincere hope that you will read this book from cover to cover, share it with your loved ones and friends, and use it often as a reference to gain control of your health by employing Dr. LaFarra's techniques.

In Balanced Health,
Dr. M. Samm Pryce

INTRODUCTION

Learning to cope with change is often a process that involves many layers of adaptation over the course of time. Change must not only occur if we are to move forward, but we must also be willing to embrace it if we are to create the best environment to promote a healthy body. The past fifteen years have come and gone with numerous life lessons that reminded me I wasn't prepared to deal with or manage stress, and I needed to make changes to find my best health. I realized I was lost and lacked the knowledge to deal with my issues, so I desired to have a healthy life and I sought resources to assist me in doing so. There is so much more to learn about being healthy than drinking water and avoiding red meats.

As a teenager, I was diagnosed with an autoimmune disease. My childhood was hindered by the physical limitations caused by this disease. At times, I had to push myself beyond the norm and more often to physical and mental extremes as I achieved each new academic milestone from student to physician. I suffered from sleep deprivation and physical exhaustion as I obsessed over ways to fit in rather than stand out, except academically because I felt this part of my life was so much easier to control. All of this was silently taking a toll on my health. As a result, my mind had to be recalibrated many times along this journey of becoming a medical doctor, health coach, and mother.

Looking back over the last 30 years, I have begun to appreciate the role that my ideas about food and eating have had on my state of health and even my mindset. If I had known then what I know now about how the substances I consumed either improved or aggravated my immune system, I would have definitely relied on nutrition and mindfulness to provide my body with more of the essentials for decreased inflammation.

When I decided to write this book, I decided to share the lessons I had learned over the past 10 years. This book isn't just based on my personal journey to a healthier, more productive lifestyle. It contains techniques that have also been proven to work for others that have had much success following traditional and nontraditional ways to create and maintain health. Writing this book has helped me more than I had initially realized, and I am confident that other moms can get the organization and reassurance they need to make the necessary changes in their lives and the lives of their families.

As a medical doctor, I realize that this alternative way to obtain symptomatic relief and even laboratory demonstrated cures for some individuals is not always evidence-based. However, there are some things that just can't be easily explained with a scientific study. As a patient and health coach, I have witnessed the health benefits to others who improved their health through decreasing various sources of stress.

This book is a reflection of my lifelong struggle with food we eat and food that nourishes us from outside the plate that can affect us from the outside in. Both of these can play a huge role in the development of inflammation, which leads to disease. Oftentimes, I hear parents as well as other individuals asking about ways to improve their or their children's health because of obesity, sleep issues, hyperactivity, and so on.

Traditional medical training for most physicians offers very little teaching on food as an alternative to prescribed medicine in the treatment of illness, so I found becoming a health coach a much-needed way to overcome some of the health issues I faced. My hope is that through reading this book, you will experience a little health coaching with reflections in some of the areas that have benefited me the most.

Coaching Reflection:

How have you dealt with previous disappointments, either within your career or in your personal life?

____

____

____

____

Did you feel that you had good coping mechanisms, or do you feel that you internalized negativity which could have caused health problems to develop?

____

____

____

____

What role do you feel food and eating played in dealing with unpleasant situations?

____

____

____

____

What other factors could have contributed to how you dealt with those situations?

____

____

____

____

MY STORY

Growing up in rural Mississippi as the oldest of four children, my mother played the most important role in shaping how I saw myself and the world around me. She often regretted her decision to put off finishing college, instead becoming a housewife and not the nurse she had dreamed of being. I was about six years old when I decided to make her proud by becoming a doctor since she had wanted to be a nurse, so I convinced myself to find out all the mistakes she felt she had made so I could avoid them. She returned to college as I entered high school, and I witnessed her metamorphosis into this college graduate and nurse that had gained so much confidence over the course of my high school years.

My mom's return to college began my introduction, along with my oldest brother, to the practice of cooking. It was a very memorable experience for us. We quickly learned that red beans and rice wasn't supposed to be crunchy, that salt should probably be measured if one isn't familiar with cooking, and that sandwiches were a pretty good alternative to home cooked meals. With a grandfather that was a farmer, we often had plenty of fresh seasonal vegetables, and we were kids that actually looked forward to freshly picked peas, red and green tomatoes, butterbeans, okra, corn, and peanuts. Not realizing it at the time, we ate quite a few organic vegetables. I never forgot my love for whole foods and its beginnings in my childhood.

I was about sixteen years old when I began having muscle spasms and feeling unusually fatigued, especially when I was stressed about something. It was hard to convince others of the hard time I was having because I didn't look sick most of the time. It's quite common for many who are later diagnosed with autoimmune disease to be told by others that they are hypochondriacs or are seeking attention because they don't look sick. My knuckles would turn red and swell quite often and frequently left me with sweaty hands, which got worse with anxiety, causing me to withdraw from many social interactions. I felt socially handicapped for years because I didn't want people to notice; nevertheless, I grew to accept my condition. Aside from the occasional joint aches and skin discolorations, I managed to remain flare-up free during young adulthood. I was diagnosed with a lupus-like autoimmune disease that didn't meet all of the criteria for any particular disorder. Many of my problems with my autoimmune disease resumed once I finished medical school and again when I was almost done with my four years of pathology residency.

I vividly recall the day that I passed my chairman attempting to make it outside and into my car before anyone noticed my legs were about to give out, only to find myself couch-bound and alone with my thoughts once I made it home. I couldn't walk without assistance for three days. I recovered only to develop bilateral uveitis within the next several months. It was confirmed that I had a disease called sarcoidosis, and this was the autoimmune disease that didn't fully meet all diagnostic criteria for one particular disease until now. About two years after giving birth to my twin sons, I again had terrible symptoms due to my sarcoidosis. I remember sitting at my desk at work and feeling nauseous and having pain in my side. The pain grew so intense within a matter of minutes that I found myself on the floor of my office in the doorway hoping someone would come and help me. I had to be wheeled to the emergency room by my coworkers. That day I was diagnosed with kidney stones, another manifestation of sarcoidosis. Within the course of a year, shortness of breath led to imaging that showed lymph nodes in my chest the size of golf balls (normally they are smaller than kidney beans). I did several months of che-motherapy with corticosteroids. My symptoms remained controlled for about four years until I began having prob-lems at work and home, which ended in divorce, a new job, and new living arrangements.

It was during this time that I was able to partner with a chef to open a Cajun restaurant, which I enjoyed, but it also brought along a tremendous amount of stress. I was so pleased that the food was not only savory but also afforded healthy options for those seeking that very thing when they couldn't cook at home. Symptoms of my illness again appeared, this time bringing with them an unintentional weight loss of 20 percent of my body weight and recurrent yeast infections. No matter what I tried, I couldn't gain the weight back. This is when I was fortunate enough to meet my friend and naturopathic doctor, Dr. Samm. What we came up with as a diagnosis was a little unbelievable to me even as a pathologist, but it all started to make sense. I had been exposed to mold in two of the places where I had lived within the last cou-ple of years, and my body was no longer absorbing what I ate. The night we felt certain that I had mold overgrowth causing many different symptoms was the night that tre-mendously changed my life once more. I nervously sat in my car on my speakerphone as she told me to do what I was so afraid of—I had to give up nearly everything I had been eating for the last several months to begin an Anti-Candida diet. I could no longer eat certain nuts, fruit, cheese, pastas with mushrooms, bread, and food containing yeast, among other things that I enjoyed eating.

An Anti-Candida diet is a modified form of the Paleo diet with elimination of some foods that may promote the growth of yeast and added foods thought to be anti-fungal which starve the yeast. This diet is not supported by scientific evidence, but I was willing to try anything. Meats, eggs, fish, and non-starchy vegetables along with vegetables that contain antifungal properties (garlic, coconut oil, ginger, and cinnamon) are necessary over an extended period of time to rid the body of mold and its symptoms. Anything high in sugars (many fruits) or anything that contained properties that feed fungus like peanut butter, pasta, most breads, and mushrooms was off limits. I felt so lost that evening as I strolled the aisles of Whole Foods with a grocery list of foods that I could actually eat and wondered how I was going to survive. I know this sounds a little extreme, but I honestly don't ever want to feel that way again. One of the main components of my diet over the next few months would be an early morning blend of two garlic cloves along with fresh greens and the occasional three or four blueberries when I felt as if I could no longer tolerate the garlic.

Within a matter of weeks, I was using the same lifestyle skills I had just learned to decrease stress and inflammation during my second pregnancy. I experienced no complications despite being ten years older than I was during my first pregnancy and being a high-risk patient. During my second pregnancy, my decision to eat a few more plant-based foods a day in addition to maintaining a positive mindset—no matter the situation—had surprising results. My doctors and my coworkers noticed the changes in me. The chronic significant anemia for which I had been worked up twice for genetic causes had gone away, and a few of my coworkers commented that I had more energy than I did before pregnancy. I was able to work through the last week of a healthy full-term pregnancy without any postpartum complications.

My autoimmune condition, as I have learned over the years, was multifactorial in development. I do feel that having an appreciation for whole foods at the beginning of my life helped to delay symptoms that became magnified as a young adult. My story is just one example of why we, as moms, should strive to teach our children the importance of eating a healthy and balanced diet, and healthy ways to deal with stress. My mother's home cooking and my grandfather's harvest are reminders of the great start that I was blessed with for eating whole foods and the role a strong nutritional foundation plays in delaying disease onset and progression. I am now very aware that my ability to stay away from a diet of predominantly packaged and processed foods that have been tied to the development and flare-ups of autoimmune disease likely contributed to the symptoms of my disease holding off for so many years. The ability to show gratitude for my previous experiences has also been extremely helpful in the management of my stress. I now realize that negative experiences are sometimes a part of the preparation for greater things. I will explain in more detail later how inflammation caused by external factors (which lead to stress) as well as how the foods we eat can lead to not only autoimmune diseases but also many of the other chronic diseases from which some of us suffer. My desire for the reader of this book is to increase your comfort level with having meaningful conversations with your physician and to enhance your ability to care for yourself and those you love.

Chews #1:

Identify Two Events From Your Past That Have Had the Most Influence on Your Present Concept of Health:

1. _______________________________________

____

____

____

2. _______________________________________

____

____

____

THE LINK BETWEEN CHRONIC INFLAMMATION AND COMMON DISEASES

The Impact of Chronic Diseases on Your Health

Chronic disease is a general terminology describing any disease that persists for at least one year and causes limitations in physical activity, ongoing medical activity, or both. Chronic diseases are time-consuming and economically costly, comprising the majority of the health care expenditures in this country. According to the CDC, six out of ten adults in the United States have a chronic disease, and four out of ten adults have at least two. The list of chronic diseases consists of: cancer, heart disease and its complications, autoimmune diseases, obesity, skin problems such as eczema, and dementia, just to name a few. Many symptoms are well characterized while others are vague such as insomnia, fatigue or difficulty concentrating. As previously mentioned, the majority of chronic diseases have a component of inflammation, which can be seen outwardly in such ways as redness and swelling or inwardly as it leads to disease processes when chronically present.

Inflammation, a response or process in the body resulting in redness, swelling, and pain is often a reaction to injury or infection. A major role of inflammation is to protect our bodies by mounting immune responses against harmful viruses, bacteria, fungi, parasites, and other pathogens. Our white blood cells along with some other cells in our immune system (e.g., macrophages) are the soldiers in this fight against foreign invaders into our bodies. In some cases, our immune system begins an inflammatory response against the tissues and organs in our own body. For instance, the joints are affected in rheumatoid arthritis; white matter in the brain and spinal cord of multiple sclerosis; lymphoid tissue, skin, lungs, and eyes in sarcoidosis; gut in celiac disease and Crohn's disease; thyroid gland in Hashimoto's Thyroiditis or Graves' disease; kidneys, skin, and various organs in lupus; and myelin of the optic nerve and spinal cord in Devic's disease. These are just a few of the many autoimmune diseases, and I have either been a part of the treatment or have known someone with each of these.

Let's take a look at some of these chronic diseases and the role of inflammation in their pathogenesis. Some of the more common inflammation related chronic diseases include: hypertension, diabetes, celiac disease, coronary artery disease, depression, Alzheimer's disease and dementia, chronic kidney disease, and arthritis. We will briefly discuss the pathogenesis (or the way the disease begins) of a few of these diseases and the role inflammation plays in causing illness.

Autoimmune Disease

The body's immune system attacks itself in an individual with autoimmune disease. Autoimmune disease often affects twice as many women as men, with some such as lupus affecting nine women to one man. Overall, the lifespan of a person with an autoimmune disease can be shortened by eight years. Though autoimmune diseases are relatively uncommon to much of the population, almost twice as many billions of dollars are spent on treatment of these diseases each year compared to cancer.

In the case of celiac sprue (or celiac disease), this type of reaction occurs when a food substance known as gluten is eaten. Symptoms range from intestinal upset, to malabsorption in the small intestine due to flattening of absorptive structures there known as villi, skin rashes, and fatigue. Treatment of sprue, like many other diseases with known causes, includes removing the offending substance from the body. In the case of sprue, a gluten-free diet is consumed. A few other well-known autoimmune conditions include: lupus, rheumatoid arthritis, multiple sclerosis, and sarcoidosis. Most of these diseases take years to diagnose due to the right mix of recognizable symptoms taking time to manifest. They also may go unrecognized, therefore preventing a specific autoantibody from being tested for in many patients. A genetic component may exist in some families containing more than one autoimmune disease but not necessarily the same disease.

Lupus is due to an unknown agent causing a flare-up within the body, which results in different body tissues coming under attack. Lupus may cause damage to organs such as the skin, kidneys, heart, lungs, muscles, and joints resulting in low-grade fever, fatigue, hair loss, and fluid accumulations known as effusions around some organs. Rheumatoid arthritis manifests as joint swelling with pain and deformity as time goes on and some skin symptoms such as nodules. Flare ups are episodes in autoimmune diseases when symptoms become worse and more noticeable. Multiple sclerosis flare ups result from autoimmune attacks on the nervous system possibly leading to fatigue, muscle spasms, blindness, and upper and lower body limb weakness. Sarcoidosis flare-ups may manifest as bilateral uveitis of the eyes, fatigue, shortness of breath with lung involvement, skin lesions known as granulomas, kidney stones, enlarged lymph nodes, and rarely sarcoid cardiomyopathy, which may result in sudden death. Most of these autoimmune diseases are treated with a course of oral steroids, sometimes intravenous steroids, and biologics, which in rare cases have been shown to cause lymphoma or other forms of cancer. The ultimate goal of all the treatments listed above is to decrease inflammation to alleviate the symptoms. Other therapies that are nonpharmaceutical include: dietary control of symptoms with diets that are anti-inflammatory, checking for hidden fungal infections or food allergens, stress management, and exercise.

Obesity

Obesity is an epidemic that has more than doubled in incidence over the last three decades with one in three adults and almost half of African Americans being overweight. According to the CDC, obesity accounts for almost 10 percent in medical spending with over $140 billion in obesity related spending in 2008. An unhealthy weight often means a greater risk for other health conditions such as type 2 diabetes, heart disease, and even many cancers.

Inflammation is absolutely a component of obesity. Based upon various studies, it seems as though obesity and inflammation feed one another in a vicious cycle. Increased adipocytes (fat cells) in the body release inflammatory substances. This can lead to chronic diseases such as metabolic syndrome, which is a precursor to diabetes and atherosclerosis.

This does not mean that all obese individuals will develop these conditions, but their chances of developing poor health outcomes are higher.

Lifestyle Modifications:

Become knowledgeable about what a healthy weight is for your height (see section below on High Body Mass Index (BMI) and Ideal Weight). If you don't see a physician regularly, seek medical approval before beginning special diets and exercise routines to ensure you are healthy enough to do so. Calculate your BMI (possibly using Google or a fitness app) to have a better perspective of your weight and its potential health effects prior to your scheduled doctor's visit.

Gut Inflammation

The gastrointestinal tract is a gateway to substances entering the body. Once in the mouth and swallowed, food and liquids begin their journey down into your gastrointestinal tract or the gut. What goes in must come out, unless it is absorbed into the body. This absorption or lack of absorption is where many illnesses begin, believe it or not. As much as 70 percent of our immune system is located in our gut, so this explains why mindfulness about what we eat is so important. A few factors including the wellness of the gut and a normal balance of gut bacteria or flora determine how our bodies will interact with what we have ingested. The gut flora normally occupies the inside of the intestine and in most cases allows digestion to proceed relatively smoothly in regular day-to-day operations, unless an overgrowth of bad bacteria occurs resulting in various symptoms such as stomach upset, obesity, autoimmune diseases, or malabsorption disorders. This state of imbalance is known as dysbiosis. "Bad" bugs may outnumber "good" bugs, which may be affected by the Western fast food diet, antibiotics, and traces of other substances found in the food we ingest. Dysbiosis may result in an inability to lose weight. Children and adults who eat diets that are high in fiber and low in processed foods and sugars have overall better gut health.

Good bacteria often help to create a happy medium that guards against inflammation and blocks harmful substances from entering the body to cause disease. A condition known as leaky gut may occur once good bacteria can no longer protect the gut lining. Leaky gut is linked to weight gain, obesity, diabetes, inflammatory bowel disease, and certain cancers. Studies have shown that one major factor that changes gut flora composition for up to four years in some individuals is taking a course of antibiotics for illness. The flora of skinny individuals continues to somehow protect them from obesity. Dietary factors in some plants known as lectins are also described as a major cause of leaky gut syndrome and disease. Lectins may prevent adequate digestion and are often in the seeds of plants such as peanuts, some beans, and corn.

Antibiotic residue is a contaminant of the water supply across the United States and is used in many products daily. Antibiotics are used in agriculture to prevent disease in overcrowded living conditions of the animals we consume.

Many diseases that involve inflammation occur in the gastrointestinal tract. Sometimes the substances we ingest such as gluten (a component found on certain grains such as wheat and barley) may cause an immune reaction with intestinal upset and malabsorption in the small intestine. Skin rashes and fatigue are among other symptoms that may occur.

Lifestyle Modifications:

Establishing a healthy balance of mixed gut flora may be needed in some individuals with difficulty losing weight, and this too can be done predominantly through the diet. A lower calorie diet is often used in such individuals. In individuals whose gut flora is dysbiotic, it is important to remember when beginning adjustment that sugar feeds the bacteria already there, which may lead to even more overgrowth, which may exacerbate a problem with inflammation. Prebiotics combined with probiotics are a good start to restoring a healthy mix of gut flora. Prebiotic carbohydrates can feed bacteria and are nondigestible fibers that can be found in foods such as raw jicama; allium vegetables such as garlic, onions, scallions, leeks, whole-grain and sprouted-grain bread, soybeans; potato skins; apple cider vinegar; avocadoes; and dandelion greens. Prebiotic foods can be eaten raw or cooked, but cooking changes the composition of the recommended 5 grams a day of the fiber. Once they pass through the upper gastrointestinal tract, they reach the colon where they are fermented by the gut flora. These are also called oligosaccharides or types of fiber. They feed the "good" bacteria such as probiotics in the colon. They help with immunity, weight control, and regularity. Probiotics (typically fermented to produce healthy bacteria) found in foods such as yogurt, cheese, sauerkraut, kimchi, beer, kombucha, kefir, and cultured butter have very different roles from prebiotics in the gut. Probiotics help to protect against harmful bacteria that causes certain types of diarrhea, help to prevent constipation, and help to strengthen the immune system. Individuals on antibiotics may often benefit from taking prebiotics afterwards to feed and repopulate "good" bacteria that may have died off. Getting enough fruits, vegetables, and other sources of fiber are likely to be helpful with gut microbiome recovery after a course of antibiotics Please keep in mind that different probiotic capsules contain different strains of bacteria that may work better in some individuals more than others, and that those used are live.

Hypertension

Hypertension or high blood pressure, the most common cause of cardiovascular risk factors leading to disease and death in our country, is a disease of the blood vessels, diagnosed when the blood pressure is greater than 130/80. Prior to 2017, this diagnosis was made when a blood pressure was 140/90. It was consistently reported in studies that individual s with high-normal blood pressure sustained damage to end organs such as the kidneys.

Essential hypertension is increasingly more common as we age. The disease process of hypertension has been demonstrated to be linked to inflammation due to a few mechanisms. Factors such as oxidative stress, activation of the sympathetic nervous system, and endothelial cell (cells lining the blood vessels) dysfunction may result from inflammation. Endothelial cells may demonstrate dysfunction in inflammation by modifying the rate of synthesis of nitric oxide (NO), a vasodilator. White blood cells have markers for stress hormones, which may be activated by the sympathetic nervous system, and oxidative stress may occur due to release of reactive oxygen species from white blood cells. Reactive oxygen species are normally released when fighting infection or foreign matter entering the body. C-reactive protein (CRP) is the proinflammatory marker seen most commonly in prehypertensive patients in some studies. Hypertension is treated with pharmaceuticals often targeting various receptors in the body.

Lifestyle Modifications:

Nonpharmaceutical therapies including controlling stress, decreasing salt intake, regular exercise or weight loss (waist circumference in men should be less than 40 inches and less than 35 inches in women), healthy eating, smoking cessation, treatment of sleep apnea, and consuming such substances as omega 3 fish oil can be implemented. Foods that lower blood pressure also include the Dietary Approach to Stop Hypertension (DASH) and the Mediterranean diet: legumes, beet juice and beet greens, kale, ground flaxseed, Swiss chard, blueberries, moringa oleifera, spinach, olive oil (polyphenols), and arugula juice. Many of these have nitrates to relax blood vessels, and foods rich in potassium such as sunflower seeds also lower blood pressure. Many of us can also appreciate the cacao in dark chocolate being on this list. These are just a few of the substances that have demonstrated the ability to lower blood pressure.

Diabetes

Diabetes is a disease of insulin resistance discussed so often in this country that it's hard to believe that most of the 300,000 undiagnosed and unaware people who have this devastating disease don't recognize their symptoms and seek treatment. Diabetes is diagnosed when a single random blood glucose is greater than 200 mg/dL, a fasting blood glucose is greater than 126 mg/dL, two oral glucose tolerance tests of 75 grams are elevated or a HbA1c (3 month average of blood sugars) is greater than six-and-a-half. There are two main types of diabetes: type 1 and type 2. Type 1 diabetes is not discussed as often as type 2 but it affects a different set of people. Type 1 diabetes is due to insulin resistance from an autoimmune attack against the cells in the pancreas that produce insulin and leads to dependence on insulin from an outside source. Type 1 diabetics are usually younger and have had some type of infection, such as strep throat, that weakens the immune system and opens the body up to attacking itself in susceptible individuals.

The big question for diabetes in this book is, "How is it related to inflammation?" Many overweight type 2 diabetics have chronic low-grade inflammation. Inflammation and stress responses are linked to insulin resistance.

The devastating complications of type 2 diabetes can be prevented by knowing some of the risk factors such as overweight habitus; family history; prediabetes; high level of cholesterol or triglycerides or low HDL; certain ancestries (African American, Pacific Islander, Native American, Hispanic or Latino); having gestational diabetes; birthing a baby weighing more than nine pounds; age older than 45 years; or, having polycystic ovarian syndrome. If you have developed diabetes, taking control of glucose levels will decrease the following symptoms: increased hunger, increased thirst, increased urination, unexplained weight loss, fatigue, numbness in the hands and feet. Though these symptoms may be present and lead a doctor to perform a diagnostic test, other people may not find out they have diabetes until they have evidence of organ damage such as heart disease.

Lifestyle Modifications:

I like to use an acronym called L.E.A.P. for diabetes prevention:

1. **Lose** approximately 5 percent of body weight (a 200-pound person who loses 10 pounds) to increase insulin sensitivity because increased body fat desensitizes

cells to insulin. This can be done by cutting back on calories or increasing physical activity to at least 30 minutes a day of brisk walking for three to five times a week.

2. **Eat** a balanced diet with healthy portion sizes and amounts (five to nine servings of fruit and veggies a day along with three servings of whole grains). Maintain a diet with a low glycemic index as this also helps to decrease low-grade chronic inflammation and the risk of metabolic syndrome. Fiber in different fruits and vegetables decreases blood sugar. Moringa leaf powder has been shown in some studies to reduce blood sugar by over 10 percent and over 20 percent in some.

   Home cooking is a great idea as you have a lot more control over what enters your body.

3. **Avoid** sweet drinks and diet sodas while adding an accountability partner to keep you motivated.

4. **Physical** activity increases as you develop habits such as turning the TV off, dancing, or starting a morning exercise routine.

These changes are ways to increase insulin sensitivity in type 2 diabetes and decrease the levels of chronic inflammation in the body.

Depression

Depression is clinically diagnosed when five or more diagnostic criteria for major depressive disorder (such as depressed mood, changes in appetite or weight, insomnia, fatigue, or feelings of guilt or worthlessness) are met within the same two weeks. At least one of these symptoms must be depressed mood or loss of interest or pleasure. Chronic conditions associated with stress (e.g., heart disease, diabetes, multiple sclerosis, and autoimmune diseases) are usually more common in those with depression.

Lifestyle Modifications:

A few ways to combat depression include decreasing inflammation by activities such as eating healthier and avoiding foods with high sugar content such as soda, white bread, and pastries along with margarine, lard, fried foods, and red meat. Consumption of anti-inflammatory foods such as tomatoes, green leafy vegetables, walnuts, fish, berries, and plant oils such as olive oils also help with depression symptoms. Other inflammation fighting activities include mental exercises such as deep breathing or yoga and regular physical exercise.

Coaching Reflection:

Do you or your children struggle with chronic diseases that increase inflammation within your body?

____

____

____

____

How important is it to you to learn ways to decrease inflammation and create a more energized and possibly happier life?

____

____

____

____

Other Indicators of Chronic Disease Explained: Abnormal HDL, LDL, Cholesterol, and Triglycerides

Do you know what happens to fat once your body breaks it down inside the gut? The body can get energy from dietary fats, fats that are stored, and through biosynthesis from carbohydrates such as glucose. Fats mostly come from animal sources, but fat or lipid metabolism also occurs in plants. Most of the fat we take into the body ends up as triglycerides, which consist of three fatty acid molecules attached to glycerol. Triglycerides are broken down into a monoglyceride and free fatty acids are absorbed into the intestine, recombine into triglyceride once they exit the intestinal lining, and combine with cholesterol and special proteins called lipoproteins.

Lipoproteins are named according to their density levels and consist of LDL cholesterol, VLDL cholesterol, and HDL cholesterol. Cholesterol is carried from the liver by LDL, which participates in the formation of atherosclerosis (precursor to hardened and clogged vessels). HDL carries cholesterol from the liver for excretion into the gut or to the other tissues or for hormone production in other tissues. Cholesterol and triglyceride levels become risk factors for heart disease when the total cholesterol is greater than 200 mg/dL and triglycerides are greater than 150 mg/dL. It becomes a little easier to see why some refer to LDL as the bad cholesterol and HDL as the good cholesterol based on their roles in the body.

As good cholesterol, the HDL molecule takes cholesterol to the liver where it can be eliminated from the body instead of building disease in vessels. HDL ranges from less than 40 mg/dL (risk factor for cardiovascular diseases), to 40 mg/dL to 60 mg/dL (decreases risk factor for cardiovascular disease), to HDL greater than 60 mg/dL (considered protective against heart disease).

Lifestyle Modifications:

HDL can be raised or lowered by certain habits such as exercise consisting of at least 30 minutes of moderate activity at least three days a week. A healthy diet high in saturated fats in oils from foods such as avocado, coconut, nuts, and olive oils, limiting exposure to smoking—even second-hand—and less than moderate alcohol consumption (one drink a day for women and two drinks a day for men).

HDL may be lowered by decreasing intake of processed foods, margarine, fried foods, and shortening. The FDA has enforced strict regulations to limit detrimental health effects due to trans fats and hydrogenated oils, originally used to enhance taste. LDL cholesterol greater than 160 mg/dL is considered high and a risk factor for heart disease. LDL can be lowered by eating soluble fibers present in some whole grains, fruits, and vegetables.

Elevated Glucose (High Blood Sugar)

Glucose is one of the simple building blocks that the body breaks down complex carbohydrates into for energy. Normal amounts of glucose include a fasting glucose usually between 70 mg/dL and 100 mg/dL. When glucose levels are abnormally elevated, particularly for extended periods of time, a diagnosis of diabetes or prediabetes is considered as described in the above paragraphs about diabetes.

Lifestyle Modifications:

Blood glucose can be lowered by eating soluble fibers such as those present in the bran layer of some whole grains, fruits, and vegetables. The risk of developing type 2 diabetes can also be reduced with measures that decrease blood glucose. Consuming a diet rich in foods with a low glycemic index, or a slow rate of metabolizing carbohydrates, raises blood sugar more slowly and assists in providing better control of diabetes symptoms.

High Blood Pressure

An individual's blood pressure is determined by the force exerted by the blood on the blood vessels as the heart contracts and relaxes between contractions. Blood pressure measurement is taken by a cuff that measures pressure mostly over the brachial artery or over the femoral artery in the leg. The blood pressure measurement consists of two numbers: systolic pressure and diastolic pressure. The systolic pressure is the top number and the diastolic pressure is the bottom number. Both numbers are measured in millimeters of mercury (mmHg).

A normal blood pressure is optimal for good vascular function and protects against damage to the vessel wall caused by high blood pressure. A normal blood pressure is less than 130/80. Prior to 2017, a diagnosis of hypertension or high blood pressure was made when a blood pressure was over 140/90. It was consistently reported in scientific studies that individuals with high-normal blood pressure sustained damage to end organs such as the kidneys, blood vessels in the eyes and brain leading to kidney failure, possible blindness, and nervous system diseases such as stroke and dementia. Blood pressure that is not well-controlled can be due to a variety of factors such as hormonal, diet-induced, and genetic predisposition to the condition. Another factor that is less mentioned but probably plays a larger role than previously discussed in many cases is just what you guessed… inflammation.

Lifestyle changes such as decreased sodium consumption as in the DASH diet, decreased alcohol consumption, smoking cessation, weight loss, low-calorie healthy diets, and regular physical activity either prevent or reverse symptoms in some cases.

High Body Mass Index (BMI) and Ideal Weight

Have you ever heard someone share their weight and feel like you were doing such a poor job of managing your own health because your numbers were nowhere close to that other person's? If this has happened to you, did you note the other person's height or whether either of you work out? There are likely a few problems with the comparison that you made—a proper comparison of weight can only be made taking other factors, not just a single number, into account. A health parameter known as body mass index (BMI) does just that.

BMI is a number often used to standardize your body habitus in relation to others based on your height and weight, allowing professionals to discuss possible body fat in easily understood numbers. It gives a general idea as a screening measurement of the amount of body fat, bone, and muscle in an individual. An adult individual with a BMI of less than 18.5 kg/m2 is considered underweight, 18.5 to 25 is normal, 25 to 30 is overweight, and over 30 kg/m2 is obese. A child's BMI is expressed as a percentile based on age and sex for children and teens two to twenty years old. A BMI less than the 5th percentile is underweight, the 5th percentile to less than the 85th percentile is normal, the 85th to the 95th percentile is overweight, and equal to or greater than the 95th percentile is obese.

Like weight, a BMI alone does not determine a patient's health status without taking other factors such as physical activity and muscle mass, body fat measurement, and waist circumference into consideration. Would you expect a muscular professional athlete with a BMI of 25 to have the same risk factors for chronic disease as an inactive individual with the same BMI? Certainly not. Here's why. Assigning a diagnosis of overweight based solely on a number would place the same athlete with low triglycerides, a normal to high HDL, and minimal body fat into the same disease risk category as the naturally thin inactive person if decisions were made based on only one or two health parameters. A recent study discussed on a blog I contributed to on myfitnesspal.com confirmed that increased weight and BMI both conferred a higher cardio-vascular risk even with other measurable risk factors being normal. Therefore, they should still get regular checkups.

"So, what is my ideal weight?" Honestly, the answer depends on the individual and a truthful assessment of many factors such as family genetics, an individual's health status, the diet or eating lifestyle they are willing to adopt, and even an individual's recommended numbers such as BMI, triglycerides, and blood pressure. The ultimate answer for the ideal weight comes down to being as close as possible to a normal weight and BMI through lifestyle changes that allow for normal cardio-vascular risk factors (verified by regular doctor's visits). A discrete number for ideal weight can be reached using the Hamwi equation. For women: one hundred pounds plus five pounds for each inch over five feet, and minus five pounds for each inch under five feet. For men: one hundred and six pounds plus six pounds for each inch over five feet, and minus six pounds for each inch under five feet. Weights within 10 percent of this equation are within normal limits.

Young Parental Age When Chronic Disease Developed

As the lifespan of the population increases, the possibility of developing certain heritable diseases is greater. My family history of hypertension, diabetes, and rheumatoid arthritis caused me to rethink my lifestyle as a whole. I would use this new concept of food as medicine to counteract the changes in my body that caused my immune system to fight against me. As a physician, I am taught that diseases manifest through a complex interaction of nurture versus nature. My genes don't make me, they just provide a map that my body along with my environment can choose to adhere strictly to or not. I am a combination of every internal and external factor that has occurred in my life. Every aspect of my life was up for reflection as I wondered where I went wrong and what caused disease to catch up with me. Why was I the only one in my family with lymph nodes in my chest the size of golf balls and the "Batman X-ray" as my doctors put it? Or, was I?

About 40 years later in life than me, my mother was also diagnosed with sarcoidosis. Her symptoms were much milder than mine, and she is now disease and medication free. Her disease presented itself totally different from mine except for one thing... the lymph nodes. Her chest lymphadenopathy caused pressure on some of her larger blood vessels, leading to swelling of just one of her legs for years. Our ages were not helpful since I was much younger when I was diagnosed, but there are many other chronic diseases that can be diagnosed or suspected spot on because of a person's relative having the same disease at a very similar age with very similar symptoms.

There are stories like these in many families to support the need for a good family history when taking a medical history. Although genetics are particularly strong, there are ways of changing one's environmental factors to delay and possibly prevent onset of chronic disease. An overweight individual with two diabetic parents, who is almost the same age his parents were when they became ill, should not take science for granted. Regular doctor's office visits for blood chemistries, including glucose and A1C, should not be avoided. Daily sodas and candy bars should not be staples in your diet. Memory difficulties should not be ignored in a 50-year-old whose parent was diagnosed with Alzheimer's disease, and this should be discussed with a physician. We can't change which family we were born into and what we are more likely at risk to develop, but we CAN alter our course. I have read about and even seen individuals who eliminate chronic diseases through lifestyle changes.

Chews #2:
Identify Two Potential Manifestations of
Inflammation in Your Life:

1. _______________________________________

____

____

____

2. _______________________________________

____

____

____

HEALTH COACH—A NEW PLAYER ON THE HEALTHCARE TEAM

Most of us are familiar with the usual health care providers such as doctors, nurses, and mental health counselors that help us to achieve better health. Conventional medicine has made great advances over the past hundred years, and many of us either have benefited personally or know someone who relies regularly on medications to control the symptoms of various diseases. As a pathologist, I am in a unique position to view disease (such as a fatty streak in a young person snowballing into an atherosclerotic plaque and a clogged heart vessel with the accumulation of additional inflammation and fat over time) microscopically in different patients from the beginning to the end of a disease process. From my perspective, it's easy to make the connection of losing inflammation to correcting a disease. I am proud to be trained as a provider of conventional medicine, which is a dynamic field continuously improving the quality of life for so many of us. I can remember having a small peppering of courses throughout my four years of medical school that provided opportunities to present information regarding various preventative health topics such as smoking cessation or the effects of tanning beds on skin cancer, but only an occasional course touched on nutrition and the healing properties of food.

This was almost twenty years ago, and my profession has made leaps and bounds with the addition of several who are a new breed of doctors who treat the whole person with specialization in a variety of lifestyle modifications using both preventative as well as conventional therapies that provide relief from many of the illnesses that ail us. These treatments get to the root of the problem instead of just treating symptoms once they have begun. These functional medicine doctors or lifestyle medicine doctors form the much-needed bridge over a rift between conventional medicine and less traditional (often natural) practices such as dietary changes that sometimes even reverse chronic diseases. This small number of doctors not only prescribe medicines to treat illness, but they also counsel on diet, hygiene, and preventative measures to provide individualized treatment plans.

Health coaches, individuals who have special training to treat the underlying cause of disease by allowing the client to guide them to an individualized care plan, also assess the different aspects of lifestyle to make life-changing recommendations. Health coaches work as individual or group lifestyle coaches, as speakers, with personal trainers, and even in doctor's offices to help provide more individualized therapy to patients such as meal plans specific to disease. Health coaches often have a great deal more time than medical doctors to provide a deeper more personalized solution to their client's problems because they are often able to consistently provide half an hour or more of their time to an individual versus the limited time that can consistently be provided to patients at repeat visits. Health coaches also provide therapies similar to those of a therapist or counselor and often are able to uncover some subconscious or minimized reason for certain symptoms. Health coaches can be encountered working in various environments but often work in conjunction with other professionals from functional medicine doctors to fitness instructors and gyms. The list of health conditions that have been improved as a result of this integrative or functional medicine (combining conventional with alternative medical treatments), include: allergies, autoimmune disorders, cardiovascular disease, obesity, and fibromyalgia to name a few.

Over the past year, I have personally gained more insight into and relied heavily upon the teachings and practices of health coaching using food as medicine as well as other nonpharmaceutical ways to reduce stress to restore my body to a state of no to minimal inflammation. One of the many benefits of becoming a health coach was using this very new field to balance many areas in my life that would soon become useful in the management of my clients. The longer I studied to become an Integrative Nutrition Health Coach, focusing on the roles of nutrition and lifestyle referred to as secondary and primary foods, the more I have become able to adjust my eating habits and lifestyle practices such as meditation and self-care to assist in my journey to better health for myself and my family. I developed an appreciation for the field of health coaching because of the emphasis on combining an individual's self-awareness about lifestyle choices with their actual overall well-being, without using prescribed medicine to eliminate symptoms. Practices such as intermittent fasting, cleanses and elimination diets, bone broth fasting, and various diets such as ketogenic, plant-based, Paleo, and blood type, may complement or replace conventional medical treatments to help to transform health, often visibly reversing some health conditions.

Two months after I made the choice to consider another possibility for my recurrent yeast infections, malabsorption, and low energy, I began to consider the possibility that the occasional prescription antifungal wasn't going to cure me. I had been studying as a health coach for four months, and I was always amazed at how mindset and a few basic lifestyle changes to decrease stress (e.g., improving relationships and adding self-care) could **reverse** not just **treat** chronic diseases. One lecture that impressed me greatly was given by a woman with hyperthyroidism who was able to forego surgery due to the elimination of added sugars from her diet. My initial thoughts were, "This woman has no taste buds, and she obviously has a strong will with a lot of time on her hands to make such a commitment." Since then, I have either heard from or read about quite a few others with conditions from kidney failure due to autoimmune disease to decreases in the amounts of heart vessel blockage. Their changes often come after a few strict dietary and lifestyle changes such as the elimination of added sugars, processed foods, and animal proteins.

Here I was feeling so low that I might even use the word depressed to describe how hopeless I felt that this cycle of infection with fatigue, treatment, and temporary relief from infection was going on, and this woman was saying that she had cured her hyperthyroidism. Her lab values had confirmed that she was no longer in a state of autoimmunity that was causing her to have symptoms. This wasn't just a miracle, it was a woman taking charge and being an accountability partner in her own healing.

I will take healing over treatment any day, and I can get both with the help of conventional and alternative medical treatment. I was recently able to reverse my own illness caused by fungal overgrowth following treatment by my friend and naturopathic doctor, Dr. Samm, through much encouragement and a strict, unpleasant diet for a few weeks. Summarily, I had to stop eating refined sugars (hidden in many places on nutritional labels by the way), yeast and fungus like mushrooms, fruits with a higher glycemic index, white rice, dairy, and peanut butter, to name only a few. I also added probiotics, fermented foods, and a hefty morning blend of raw garlic to my diet. I could no longer ignore how sugars and substances in certain nuts and mushrooms exacerbated my condition.

I am by no means cured from making imperfect lifestyle choices, but I have at least learned how to recognize when I have not made the best decisions with my diet and my other lifestyle choices. I am appreciative for advances in both traditional and nontraditional medical practices for the contributions to my own well-being and for getting me where I needed to be in the shortest amount of time possible. Think of the only 8 percent of Americans that make resolutions to change their lifestyles each year and actually accomplish their goal. Why is that percentage so low? Because if such declarations were easy to achieve, we would have more success on our own. But when we become stuck, it is helpful to enlist the services of health professionals to provide that extra sense of accountability and guidance.

Chapter 3

EATING IN A POSTMODERN ERA— IS IT SAFE TO EAT ANYTHING ANYMORE?

"Chronic disease is a food borne illness. We ate our way into this mess, and we must eat our way out."

—Mark Hyman, MD

Many years ago, the population of the world began to expand along with concerns of impending food shortage. To ease concerns about a potential famine, farmers and the government devised new methods of plant cultivation that would increase food availability and improve food durability. Some techniques that were created to allow for a greater yield of a more abundant crop to feed our increasing population also introduced dilemmas. For instance, the use of pesticides in modern farming to decrease crop spoilage and improve plant resilience have been responsible historically for many environmental and health concerns. Some pesticides have been

51

demonstrated over time to have more carcinogenic potential than others, and the Environmental Protection Agency established regulations with safety limits for pesticide residue on the food that we eat. This is discussed briefly in the paragraphs of the section below.

Genetically modified organisms (GMOs) used in the genetic engineering of plants (GMOs) to increase crops have also long been speculated to contribute to the development of cancer in humans, but the levels have not been definitively linked to a specific cancer in humans at normal levels consumed in clinical studies. Between 80 to 90 percent of the corn produced in the United States is GMO as is about 90 percent of beet sugar, most commonly used as table sugar. Though no definitive studies have shown these chemicals to be harmful, it seems more than a coincidence that other countries that don't have the same level of industrialization as the United States report fewer autoimmune and chronic diseases.

After the industrialization of farming, certain grains underwent processing that stripped away outer bran and germ and many of the nutrients from the outer plant, leaving the endosperm of the plant which caused adverse reactions (e.g., autoimmune disease) in some humans consuming these refined grains. Other plant products such as soybeans and corn underwent genetic engineering that allowed mass production of these products, allowing for more creative ideas of food preparation and processing. The information in the two preceding paragraphs effectuates one major question: how do we decide if we are eating foods made from plants with the least potentially harmful effects on us and our loved ones?

Pesticides, GMOs, Dirty Dozen, and Clean Fifteen

The Environmental Working Group, created in 1992, produces a list each year of (nonorganic) foods highest in pesticides. The list is known as "The Dirty Dozen." Foods highest on this list consistently include: strawberries, spinach, apples, nectarines, peaches, and celery. Apples led the list until about two years ago when strawberries took over. In 2017, "The Dirty Dozen" list consisted of strawberries with 98 percent having residue of multiple pesticides. Most of the pesticides have not been associated with cancer, but a portion have been linked to cancer as well as hormonal imbalances, and reproductive and developmental damage. The level of pesticides in our foods is regulated by the Environmental Protection Agency (EPA), who has the position that the residue on foods is not too harmful to eat at this time. There is also a "Clean Fifteen" list with less than 1 percent of foods from this group showing detectable pesticides. Fruits on this list contained no more than four pesticides, often containing no more than one. Topping this list are avocados, sweet corn, pineapples, cabbages, sweet peas, onions, asparagus, mangoes, and cauliflower.

If cost is a reason for a lack of healthy and safe eating, just stay focused on eating a balanced diet consisting of recommended daily amounts from the five food groups. Also, buy organic from the "Clean Fifteen" list if you obsess over avoiding GMOs and pesticide exposure. If you cannot afford organic foods that are listed on "The Dirty Dozen" list, try farmer's markets for local seasonal foods, buy fresh frozen fruits and vegetables that are often frozen when fresh, and wash your fruits and vegetables with tap water and vinegar to remove some of the pesticide residue. Eating some fruits and vegetables, organic or not, promotes adherence to a balanced diet and is associated with better overall health.

Animal Farming and Antibiotics

Animal farming has also been affected by techniques used to provide adequate supply to feed our growing population. Mass production of meat products through overcrowding and restrictive conditions have required antibiotics and other agents shown to cause cancer at certain concentrations to be used to keep these animals alive long enough to grow and be used for consumption. Between 80 to 90 percent of all antibiotics used in this country are utilized for preserving the health of animals in farming. However, it's important to keep in mind that these labels (e.g., antibiotic-free) mean different things to different companies. For example, meat labeled antibiotic-free may be from animals given antibiotics at some point in their life cycle, even if not during the end.

With all of the changes that have occurred to our food supply within less than a century, it has often been noted that many of our grandparents would not recognize the food we eat today or have much familiarity with many of the diseases we suffer from today that are thought to be food-related. Despite eating lard and fatty foods with their meals so many years ago, many of our ancestors still managed to remain slender without all of today's chronic diseases such as obesity and autoimmune disease, especially at such early ages as seen in our population today. Many of our ancestors also raised their own animals for food, as opposed to the meat that we consume today. Considering the changes in our food supply and looking back at the relative lack of certain diseases in our predecessors, it is no surprise that food that is from organic and non-GMO plants and meat from animals that is grass-fed, antibiotic-free, free range, and organic is considered best for a body that is given a chance to grow without the effects of these outside substances.

With all of the information on pesticides, antibiotics, disease, and nutrient depletion it's very confusing when choosing what to eat and can be quite upsetting to the stomach. One thing to always keep in mind is how eating something makes you feel. Perhaps the reason for the increase in autoimmune diseases that are not seen in less developed countries and was not seen in our ancestors before the 1950s is related to what we eat; but, without solid proof over a population, dramatic change in the food made for our Western culture is bound to be slow. Other explanations such as the hygiene hypothesis suggests that vaccinations prevent an immune response to outside antigens present on germs and bugs causing certain infectious diseases among young children and increased antibiotic use and resistance both in humans and animals in developed countries may make them more susceptible to allergies and autoimmune disease, but nobody knows for sure. As far as treating symptoms of autoimmune disorders and allergies, if your body doesn't agree with something and you are able to pinpoint that with a method such as journaling or an elimination diet, it is best to avoid that food. If you can afford to eat organic, grass-fed, free range foods and manage external sources of stress, your body would likely be in optimal condition. Starvation is not an answer, and neither should be eating mindlessly without regard for a balanced diet. Smart eating is key. If your area offers farmers markets or community farms, it's a lot easier and cheaper to pick those seasonal organic fruits and vegetables or just switch up organic and nonorganic foods when and if possible.

Eating Plant-Based vs. Animal Proteins

Plant-based proteins and phytochemicals are proven to protect against chronic disease. Consuming only plant-based proteins initially requires a bit more patience and planning than a diet that consists of meat because most plant proteins do not have a good balance of essential amino acids, or those amino acids that your body cannot produce. Those not conscious of this may become deficient in certain amino acids because they are incomplete sources of protein.

Animal proteins have a more complete balance of amino acids; however, animal fats and high cholesterol are associated with increased risk of certain cancers, like breast cancer and colon cancer, especially years after consuming high fat diets long-term. Some people choosing temporary lifestyle changes in food consumption should be aware that "diets" are often unsustainable because they often don't provide all of the nutrients and vitamins needed for a balanced diet. Some diets prefer animal proteins and fats to plant-based proteins as a major calorie source of energy. Plant-based diets can actually reverse heart disease unlike those high in animal fats and proteins. This is due to an inflammatory response in the gut that occurs with meat consumption, even if the meat is fish and seafood.

As a native Southerner and a person with a chronic disease, this news about meat, in particular the fish and chicken, is quite disheartening. I have asked myself many times if I was willing to give up meat for better health. This is a very individual question, and no one can make the choice for you. As a health coach, I do recommend crowding out anything "bad" in the diet with good stuff. This way, your body doesn't go into rebellion and start craving the things you have told yourself you can no longer have. A diet consisting only of plant proteins is also likely deficient in other nutrients such as zinc, vitamin B12, vitamin D, and heme iron.

For those of us who don't think a vegan or vegetarian lifestyle is sustainable, I recommend crowding out the animal protein with an extra serving a day of plant-based protein. When choosing to replace animal proteins with plant proteins, start by going meat free during one meal one day at a time. Build meals from protein out. Consider using beans as a base and adding healthy fats such as nuts, avocados, and olive oil to ease hunger pains.

Nonetheless, the search for relatively safe food isn't as difficult as it seems. So, what exactly is healthy eating, and how do we avoid anxiety that may surface around meal time? I am going to attempt to ease the mind of anyone who is asking this question with a little advice in the following sections. The Choosemyplate.gov campaign has greatly simplified the recommended composition of our daily dietary intake. Five food groups are created and proportionally represented on a plate in the United States. The five food groups are divided into: fruits, vegetables, grains, protein, and dairy. Half of your plate should be fruits and vegetables, one-quarter should be grains, and one-quarter should be protein. Other countries may have food pyramids with the largest recommended food and portions at the base of the pyramid. If preparing your own meals from the sections below is still not an option because of time constraints or the inability to cook for various reasons (physical or otherwise), I still recommend becoming familiar with a few basic food facts to improve your chances of decreasing inflammation and avoiding chronic disease. I highly recommend a meal delivery service.

Various Diets

While training to become a health coach, it was very easy to be overwhelmed with the idea of mastering different types of diets and the thought that one of the over 100 diets available for various results (everything from losing weight to alleviating symptoms of disease) would become something that we could recommend to our clients.

In the past, the average individual started a particular diet because they desired to lose weight. But diets are increasingly becoming more common in a second population with various chronic diseases who wish to eliminate or decrease their symptoms and therefore their need for medications. It is always a great idea to run extreme changes in caloric intake or changes in food types by a physician who may possibly refer you to a health coach, nutritionist, or dietician for reasons such as ensuring that you are maintaining a balanced diet. A deficiency in needed vitamins, minerals, and substances often does more harm to the body than good even when a desired effect such as weight loss is experienced.

To many, it seems simple ... take in fewer calories than needed for day-to-day energy expenditure to lose weight. In the case of chronic disease, the pathophysiology, or the cause, of the disease is imperative to know if a reproducible change in diet is to cause a similar effect across individuals. For example, individuals without gluten sensitivity won't experience such dramatic improvement in joint aches, rashes, gastrointestinal upset, and fogginess that someone with intolerance or sensitivity to gluten would experience. Diets that have statistically been shown to reduce disease over entire populations include the Mediterranean and DASH diets. Many studies show that these diets higher in plant-based foods and oils show health benefits such as decreased risk of cardiovascular disease, blood pressure issues, obesity, and diabetes. The DASH diet restricts sodium to less than 2,400 mg per day, while the Mediterranean diet limits red meats in addition to the added sugars and refined grains that are common restrictions in both diets. Meat is not eliminated in these diets, but it is suggested that there is moderation of the amount consumed.

Chapter 4

TWO MAJOR TYPES OF FOODS SATISFY HUNGER

A balanced diet works optimally when combined with a balanced healthy lifestyle."

—LaFarra Young, MD

As a health coach graduate of the Institute of Integrative Nutrition, I frequently speak of the environment and circumstances that affect our bodies in almost a different language than most people are accustomed. Though a little strange at first, this way of referring to foods makes sense. We are nourished by both primary (outer) and secondary (inner) foods that we take into our bodies which I will refer to as outer and inner foods, respectively, for clarity.

Outer foods nourish us from the outside-in and are not those we consume on a plate. These environmental factors are called primary foods because they affect us so immensely and satisfy an emotional hunger. If our outer foods aren't in balance, it is entirely likely that the foods we eat (inner foods) will not be digested and utilized properly by our bodies. Outer foods include: relationships, finances, education, exercise, creativity, happiness, home cooking, and home environment.

The food that we think of when we are physically hungry, inner food, gives us the nutrients and a physical sense of satiety after eating and digestion of selections from the five food groups and even junk food. The inner food in our lives interacts with outer food to serve the purpose of nourishing the entire person from head to toe. As I gain better control over my outer foods, I continue to witness the healing powers of edible (inner) foods.

Over the past year, coaching has been invaluable for helping me to find my balance. Coaches are our own guinea pigs many times and often do not enthusiastically recommend techniques and tasks that we would not try or perform ourselves. It wasn't until I realized just how little I paid attention to what I ate on a daily basis that I began to comprehend that I was not properly nourishing my body. When assessing someone's foods in a coaching session, I like to start with the inner foods to get a general overview of how the individual views food. Therefore, I will begin by discussing healthy ways to view the foods that we eat.

Chapter 5

INNER FOODS FOR PHYSICAL HUNGER

How do we pick the right foods for ourselves and our families? It's important first of all to note that no one diet or style of eating will be complimentary to every individual's system. Even one individual may have different dietary needs at different times in their lives. What we eat may be influenced by our age, culture, state of health, and even our cravings. When it comes to our children, we hold the powerful position of influencing a large part of the relationship they will have with food. If our goals align with simply being healthy with no special restrictions, we can often consume the same diet as the rest of the family with a few differences in macronutrient requirements or portion sizes. In terms of the way we plan to eat to live and to be healthy, let's start with some of the basics: food groups and caloric needs.

Self-Assessment: Wheel of Wellness

Wheel of Wellness

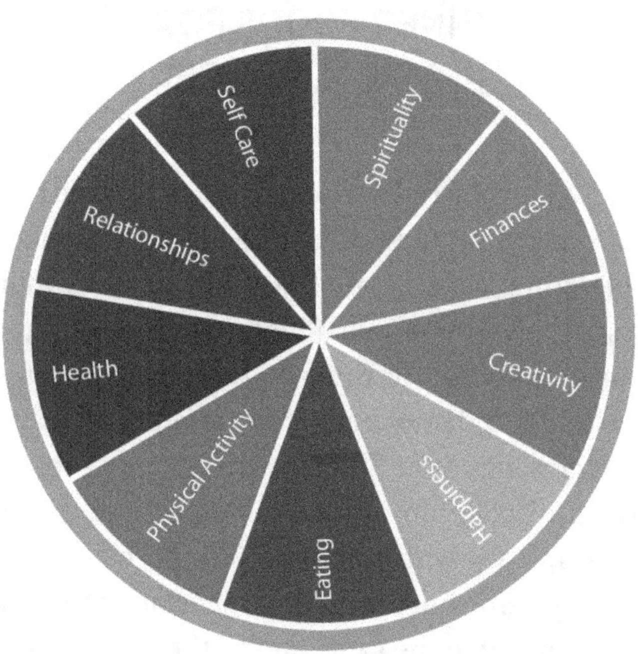

Is there balance between the critical areas in YOUR life?

1. Place a dot on each area in the wheel. The closer the dot is to the center, the more dissatisfied you are. Many people fall about halfway within each area, which is about average.

2. Connect the dots to assess your wheel for balance.

3. The areas that fall below the others indicate areas of imbalance where you should devote more time.

4. The closer your lines are to the shape of a circle, the more balance you demonstrate in your life.

Food Groups

Here are some easy guidelines regarding choosing from each group:

1. Fruits, Vegetables: provide a variety (colors of the rainbow) of vegetables and fruits for a variety of nutrients

2. Breads, Whole-grain products: 50 percent of grains should be whole grains

3. Milk, Dairy: provide nonfat or low fat milk or dairy products

4. Proteins: provide lean meats, poultry, fish, beans, and lentils

Choose appropriate portions from each food group to eat at one time and use a manufacturer's suggestion for serving size and nutritional values when purchasing processed, non-whole foods. Based on combined recommendations from the USDA and the American Heart Association recommendations, the serving sizes for the food groups are as follows:

Food Group	Number of Servings	Serving Size	Hand visual*
Grains	6-11	1 slice of bread, ½ cup of pasta (cooked), ½ bagel	Cupped hand (inside)
Fruits	2-4	1 small piece of fruit, 1 wedge of melon, ¼ cup of fruit juice, ¼ cup of dried fruit	Fist
Vegetables	3-5	½ cup of cooked beans or peas or 1 cup of chopped raw leafy greens, ¼ cup of vegetable juice	Cupped hand (cooked) or two hands (if raw leafy)
Dairy	2-3	1 cup of milk or yogurt, 1 ounce of cheese	Thumb
Protein	2-3	1 ounce chicken breast or meat, 1 egg, ½ cup cooked beans/legumes, ½ ounce nuts and seeds	Width of palm and thickness of thumb

*Hand visuals or fist symbols are also widely used to help with visualization.

NOTE: Snacks such as dried fruit and nuts have smaller serving sizes and contain more calories.

Crowding Out the Bad with Pantry and Kitchen Staples

It may seem like a lot to take in but preparing for healthy eating gets easier with time. In just months, I have progressed from mindless eating to meals that meet my nutritional needs. We particularly have to be careful, even with prepared fruits and vegetables, about the amount of added sugars we allow into our children's diets. The major sources of added sugars in American diets are regular soft drinks, sugars, candy, cakes, cookies, pies, and fruit drinks (fruit ades and fruit punch). Even dairy and milk products (ice cream, sweetened yogurt, and sweetened milk) contain these sugars. In addition, some of the obvious sources are breads and grains (i.e., cinnamon toast and honey nut waffles). The key to meal and food selection for our families is to be informed and vigilant when necessary to keep the caloric intake under a certain level.

I have the following suggestions for some relatively simple ways to **increase the nutritional content** in the meals you make for your families.

- Make your plate as <u>colorful</u> as possible. Different colors for fruits and vegetables usually suggest different nutritional benefits. For instance, purple and deep red indicates antioxidant-rich anthocyanins which decrease inflammation, and fight cancer and heart disease.

- Frozen and low sodium canned foods provide flavor and nutritional value when fresh is not available. Farmer's markets usually have locally grown seasonal vegetables and fruits with more nutrients than older produce, and they may even be grown organically with less pesticides and genetically modified organisms (GMOs).

- Strive for at least half of grains as <u>whole grains</u> vs. grains.

- When possible, <u>add protein (especially plant)</u> for increased calories and nutritional content by building meals around protein and eating high protein snacks such as hummus or nut butters. Stretch recipes by adding high protein vegetables or nuts and seeds. For example, I recently started adding hemp seeds to my bowl of red beans for a quick and easy way to get in more nutrition.

Doing this might tremendously decrease your desire to eat out.

- A <u>grocery list</u> and a weekly menu also limit mindless eating and eating out.

- <u>Added sugars</u> are not always easy to avoid. But it is much easier to detect them once you recognize that foods ending in -ose (i.e., sucrose and glucose) indicate types of sugar.

- Make water your chosen beverage, and cut back on beverages with added sugars. Water aids in digestion, flushes out toxins, prevents dehydration, and has many other health benefits.

- Stock up on <u>pantry and kitchen staples</u> for a whole food diet:

  Note: If it's not in the pantry, it cannot be consumed! Don't buy items that shouldn't be eaten at your house.

  - Pantry staples include: common nonperishable **grains** such as brown rice, wild rice, quinoa (sometimes called a seed), tortilla with tomato basil or other flour, oats, **fruit** (fresh, frozen or canned without syrup*, grapes, apples, blueberries, and oranges), **vegetables** such as chickpeas, squash, kale, cream of mushroom, spinach, black beans, green beans, carrots, and minced garlic. Low sodium and no added sugar canned vegetables and fruits are optimal.

- Staple **seasonings** include: lemon pepper, Cajun (Tony's, Old Bay, etc.), curry, cumin, rosemary, thyme, sea salt, pepper, cayenne, and cinnamon

- **Meats** include: ground turkey, organic chicken* (if possible), grass fed beef (if possible), chicken stock, fish (i.e., salmon and cod), shrimp (20/25), and crawfish. If you are going to eat meat, choose lean cuts to minimize risks associated with unhealthy fats and consume more plant proteins as part of the 25 percent recommended daily servings of proteins by dietary guidelines.

- Dairy (if desired): 2% milk, shredded natural cheese (Cheddar)

- On Fridays, gather your thoughts about what you can and will eat the following week and plan meals using what you already have available. Sometimes I prefer free apps such as MyFitnessPal and Tasty when I want to try something different.

- Fresh fruits lose much of their vitamin C content after a few days, but some canned fruit can retain vitamin C for months.

Decoding Cravings

I am often asked by various people about how to control cravings, and this prompted me to eventually give a talk solely about cravings. The talk did contain humor, but to some it's a matter of several pounds versus knowing how to say no. I will now attempt, with those who suffer in mind, to explain certain cravings.

A craving is a strong psychological desire to do something as opposed to a need to do something. During a craving, three regions of the brain are activated: hippocampus, insula, and caudate. These areas are involved in memory as well as emotional needs with hormones released due to fat and sugar that may cause a calming effect. How do you know you're craving food? In many cases, we are craving not because we are hungry but because of feelings or memories.

Some commonly craved substances are listed below with popular explanations for those cravings:

Salt: You need more water (which salt helps you to retain) because you're losing it.

Ice and inedible items such as clay, dirt, and paper with no nutritional value: You're anemic or your body is trying to increase your alertness.

Chocolate: You need love, you're getting your period, you're pregnant, or perhaps your diet is too restrictive and you are calorie or nutrient deficient.

Sweets, Carbs: You're prediabetic, you're pregnant, you're getting period, You're eating too much processed carbs, you're stressed.

Ice cream: You need soothing due to heartburn or too many pain relievers. You're tired and you need a boost of energy.

Crunchy foods: You've been eating too many soft foods or you need attention.

Steak, Burgers: You have an iron or vitamin B deficiency, or you haven't been getting enough protein.

In general, with relation to bodily functions, cravings occur because of:

1. Lack of satisfaction in an area of life. A solution is to support mind and body by working through the cause of stress.

2. Seasonal reaction: A cold person may crave warm food. Christmas cookies may be craved around Christmas time.

3. Lack of nutrients such as iron (may cause cravings for meat and cheese), magnesium (may cause cravings for chocolate), sodium (may cause cravings for salty foods, too much salt in diet).

4. Hormonal shifts: Decreased estrogen or increased progesterone may cause cravings for chocolate, sweets, and salty foods.

Here are some suggestions to deal with cravings:

1. Journal your feelings during the time of a particular craving.

2. Get a massage or a pedicure or listen to soothing music.

3. Use grounding essential oils such as sandalwood, grapefruit, and lemon.

4. Don't allow yourself to get too hungry in between meals.

5. Get seven to nine hours of sleep.

6. Prepare your food (whole grains, fruits, and vegetables) ahead of time.

7. Take longer to eat your food and chew more (chew each bite at least 10 times).

8. Gross yourself out by learning about ingredients in foods so that maybe you will no longer desire to eat them.

9. Practice portion control.

10. Prepare your own "healthy" version of the food you crave, and be mindful to avoid overeating.

Calories and Nutrition Facts Labels

Calories are the units of energy used to calculate grams of macronutrients (carbohydrates, proteins, and fats) in foods. Each macronutrient contains a certain number of calories per gram (carbohydrates have four calories, fats have nine calories, and protein has four calories). Each healthy woman and man needs between 13 and 18 calories per day per pound of body weight or 1,600 to 2,000 calories according to the 2015 Dietary Guidelines for Americans, with a normal amount of calories per day if weight loss is desired between 1,200 and 1,600 calories. Our children, beginning around four years of age, need approximately 1,200 calories per day for normal growth and development. Each child may begin to require more calories per day at differing times depending on their stature and energy requirements. Also, our children's nutritional needs often differ significantly from ours. Depending on their developmental stage, children may need more of certain nutrients than we do. Calories can be calculated using a knowledge of macronutrient content (often listed on label) or using a calorimeter. Also, for weight loss, using more energy than you take in is important.

Consuming whole foods without packaging and nutrition facts labels is recommended and often decreases the need for strict monitoring of calories. However, if you do choose packaged foods, the nutrition facts label will give you a good idea of how many calories the item contains and a breakdown of macronutrients within about a 20 percent margin of error. When looking at the nutrition facts label, it is a good idea to first note the number of calories (or grams) per serving and how many servings per package. Snack items higher than 400 calories are usually considered high in calories if you are on an 1,800-2,000 calories a day diet. Further reading details the items we need to limit, such as saturated and trans fats and sodium, followed by some of the nutrients we should try to consume enough of, such as fiber, vitamins, and minerals. Trans fats and saturated fats should be replaced with healthier fats such as polyunsaturated fats, which could help lower blood pressure. Avoid foods containing partially hydrogenated oils to decrease trans fats. One of the last items on the label is the percent daily value in a 2,000-calorie diet. When available, a footnote describes if the values for macronutrients is the higher limit for the amount in a day or if the amount listed is at least the amount needed in a day. In general, a 5 percent constitution of a nutrient is considered low and a 20 percent constitution is considered high. These cut-offs can be used when comparing two similar items to decide which to purchase or consume.

In addition to looking at nutrition facts labels, it is a good idea to read the ingredients label to find out the items used to prepare your food. A complicated ingredients label is a good indication that the food is further from the natural source and required more processing. If you can't pronounce an ingredient or recognize a whole food source, it is probably highly processed and has minimal to no nutritional value.

Once we establish where we want our family to be in terms of caloric intake and we have a general idea of our options, we could also consider the different cultural styles of food preparation and even diets that we are curious about following.

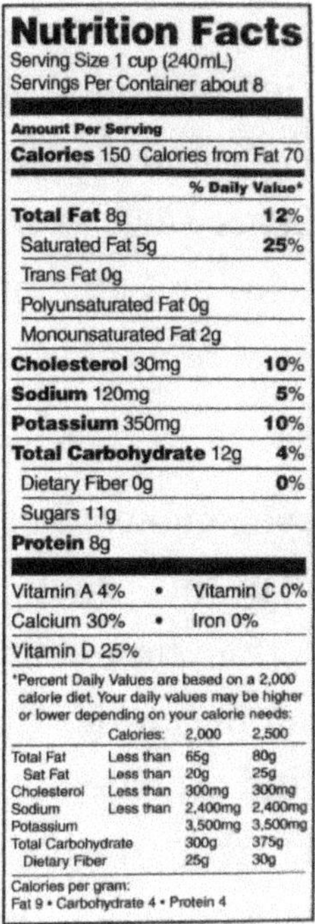

The label above is an example of an uncomplicated nutrition label. If you eat the entire packaged contents, you will consume 1,200 calories (150 calories x 8 servings) and exceed the recommended daily intake of nutrients like saturated fat and rapidly approach the limits for others like cholesterol

Another way to overcome the anxiety of whether we are meeting our nutritional needs or not is to familiarize ourselves with certain nutrient-dense foods in the various food groups.

- Grains: A variety of grains such as quinoa, brown or jasmine rice, and whole wheat can provide various nutrients such as B vitamins (folate, riboflavin, niacin, and thiamine), minerals (iron, magnesium, and selenium), and fiber.

- Vegetables:
  - Starchy vegetables: Potatoes, corn, squash, and peas in this group provide more carbohydrates than non-starchy vegetables. They are denser in calories than non-starchy vegetables and provide fiber which helps eliminate waste from the body and regulate blood sugar and cholesterol levels. These are rich

in antioxidants (beta-carotene, vitamin C, lutein, etc.), B vitamins (especially folate and B-6 which guard against memory loss, heart attack, and stroke), and minerals (potassium, magnesium, and others lower blood pressure and regulate bone health).

- Non-starchy vegetables: Broccoli, spinach, tomatoes, and peppers in this group provide fiber, potassium, vitamin K, and folate (among other vitamins and minerals). These vegetables contain about a third fewer calories and carbs than starchy vegetables.

- Fruits: Various fruits provide soluble and insoluble fibers just like vegetables. One thing to watch for with these is the amount of sugars (even though they are natural) that can be consumed, especially in the dried fruits.

- Protein: Meats as well as vegetables such as legumes contain minerals such as zinc and iron.

- Dairy: Choose low-fat or non-fat options to decrease the consumption of saturated fats. Dairy is a good source of calcium and vitamin D in children and is important for strong bones; however, many debate the need for milk as we get older in age due to the lack of lactase in many adults as well as the lack of scientific evidence of decreased fractures in adults that continue to drink milk. Many adults who are lactose intolerant have better luck with fermented milk products such as cheese.

A Simple, Balanced Low-Calorie Meal

Roast Turkey Sandwich with 1 cup of fresh fruit

Grain	Vegetable	Fruit	Protein	Dairy
Bread	2 slices of tomatoes, 1 leaf of lettuce	½ cup of apples, grapes, strawberries	Roasted turkey	Cheddar cheese
2 servings	1 serving	2 servings	2 servings	2 servings
140 calories	6 calories	60 calories	90 calories	100 calories

I'm sure we are all now a little more familiar with the five food groups and have a general idea of which foods can be found in each group. What we do with that knowledge in terms of making it practical for our families and our lifestyles is where the challenge comes in for many people. In general, a diet weighted towards whole foods is more likely to result in optimal health than a diet with too many processed foods. If you aren't meeting the daily recommendations for each food group, be conscious and plan to do better. Ninety percent of us don't get the daily recommended amounts of fruits and vegetables, so most of us have some improvements to make.

Portion Distortion

Also, avoid portion distortion, which is eating more than the recommended number of calories because the listed serving size is often smaller (kind of deceiving) than the portion size we would normally eat. Many times in restaurants, portion sizes are at least twice as large as recommended serving sizes, so it is a good idea to get familiar with normal serving sizes. For instance, a large order of fries may contain one thousand calories. Portion distortion can be reduced with a few of these practices:

- Use fist symbols of portion sizes as shown on some food pyramids to keep food portions smaller than the size of your fist. Compare your fist to the size of a measuring cup to reference serving sizes.

- Read labels carefully and adjust your portion with serving size information. If a package has 100 calories per serving with a total of two-and-a-half servings per package, your total calories will be 250 once you eat the entire package.

- Adjust your portion size to marketplace portions. If you eat an entire shake with two cups of yogurt in the ingredients, you have had two servings of dairy for the day.

- Share appetizers with others in your party to increase room for the main course.

- If the main course is large, divide it into smaller portions and take some home for leftovers.

- Use a smaller plate at home to give the perception of a larger meal.

- Eat on smaller plates.

- Add more vegetables to crowd out higher calories foods.

- Eat slowly to give your brain a chance to catch up to your stomach.

- Measure your food until you get used to portion sizes. I actually bought a small scale to keep in my kitchen to help with this.

Macronutrients

One of the greatest challenges I faced when determining the benefits of what I ate was tracking nutritional content. I was doing what I call mindless eating with no idea where I was nutritionally. Counting calories gives little value of nutritional content and provides limited information if macronutrients are not considered when trying to follow a specific diet.

The three macronutrients that make up at least a portion of each of these food groups are: carbohydrates, proteins, and fats. The Institute of Medicine has established an Acceptable Macronutrient Distribution Range (AMDR) as a guide to macronutrient distribution in our diet. Carbohydrates, largely composed of sugars and some fiber, should comprise 45 to 65 percent of your daily caloric intake. Carbohydrates contain four calories per gram, with one teaspoon of sugar containing sixteen calories and four grams of carbohydrates. 32 ounces of soda can contain 28 to 36 teaspoons of sugar, equaling around a tenth of a pound. The carbohydrates here are all sugars (no dietary fibers) with no nutritional value. Healthier foods containing carbohydrates include: fruits, legumes, dairy, whole grains, nuts, and seeds.

Over 100 years ago, Americans consumed less than two pounds of different sugars per year. Now, Americans eat 22 teaspoons of sugar a day, equaling 70 pounds per person per year. The American Heart Association currently recommends women consume less than six teaspoons or twenty-four grams per day and men consume nine teaspoons or thirty-six grams per day. The standard American diet contributes to more disease and death than alcohol and tobacco combined when we consider diabetes, inflammatory diseases, cancers, heart disease, and fatty liver. Did you know that fatty liver can lead to cirrhosis and that one in four Americans has fatty liver disease? These statistics are scary and only the beginning of too much sugar in our diet. But the good news is that these statistics don't have to pertain to all of us. Different diets consumed to decrease sugar work to drastically decrease weight in some people, and diets lower in added sugars combined with the replacement by nutrient dense foods and beverages can reduce risk of coronary artery disease (CAD). For monitoring daily macronutrients in your diet, use the amount of grams listed on the nutrition facts label and consider keeping track of calories and macronutrients with apps such as MyFitnessPal, until you become comfortable tracking these on your own.

Proteins should comprise 10 to 35 percent of your diet with four calories per gram of protein. Proteins can be found in meats such as poultry, beef, and fish, as well as in seeds and nuts, legumes, dairy, eggs, and soy. Fats contain nine calories per gram and should comprise between 20 to 35 percent of your total calories per day. Fats can be found in foods such as hummus, avocadoes, fish oil, vegetable oils, seeds, and nuts. Saturated fats found in butter, shortening, fatty meats, and whole fat dairy should be limited as much as possible. A standard four ounce serving of chicken contains twenty-five grams of protein and four grams of fat.

When tracking food intake, the source of the calories is more important than the number. Consider the nutrients missed by taking in 1,600 calories a day of junk food as opposed to a balanced diet of 1,600 calories. Macronutrient ratio may also need to be adjusted depending on weight goals and a particular diet which helps to promote adherence to the diet. For instance, 50 calories of cauliflower is more filling than 50 calories of a doughnut, mostly due to the healthy helpful fiber. Many studies show that calories should be cut overall when trying to lose weight with a focus on consuming nutrient-dense foods to feel full. Foods with both high carbohydrates and fats should be minimized during dieting as they tend to stimulate the parts of the brain responsible for cravings.

The more you know about healthy eating and numbers that contribute to health, the more you can decrease your chances of low-grade inflammation and the development of chronic diseases. Chronic diseases such as obesity, depression, autoimmune disorders, and cancer are just a few of the diseases that we develop that could be mitigated by adapting an anti-inflammatory diet or way of living. The more people there are like us who are seeking a change of lifestyle to become healthier, the closer we are to eliminating a crisis in this country. According to the Center for Disease Control, about 75 percent of the money spent on health care dollars is for the chronic diseases that result from unhealthy lifestyles.

<table><tr><td>

Chews #3:

Develop a Simple Plan to Prepare and Eat More Balanced, Healthier Meals in Four Steps:

</td></tr></table>

1. List the food group(s) that you need to increase or decrease to add more balance in your weekly diet.

____

____

____

____

____

2. Develop a list of healthy recipes (start small with about two each week) that you don't find difficult to follow.

____

____

____

____

____

3. Build meals around protein and add greens with veggies. Some believe in the concept of food combining (that their foods digest better when meats and high starches aren't mixed in the same meal), but this is up to each individual as we are all different.

4. Instead of completely eliminating your favorite not-so-healthy foods, crowd the bad foods out with the good, healthier foods.

Chapter 6

OUTER FOODS FOR EMOTIONAL HUNGER

The outer foods, probably not surprising to many of us may affect our health more significantly than the inner foods discussed above. I view most of these as taking care of yourself on the outside so that you can have peace within to optimally digest your food. As discussed previously, there are many cases where those with a large amount of emotional upset can develop or exacerbate health conditions such as high blood pressure and depression. Although I will only focus on more of the outer foods that had the greatest effects on my overall improvement, it's important to keep in mind that all areas of the wheel of wellness involve a proper mindset to address issues and a plan to resolve them.

Creativity

Activating our creative energy also serves to decrease stress and inflammation that may contribute to chronic disease. Frustration that results from not being able to express ourselves can lead to somatic manifestations in our bodies such as headaches, indigestion, and even gastrointestinal disturbances. One of the times of day that we are most productive is when there are little to no people around or when there are no time expectations set for us. Many find this time to be in the mornings before dawn. How much more productive and creative could we be if we used this time to work on our businesses or plan out our day? What about developing meal plans for the next several days? Planning helps to prevent cravings and allows for adequate nutrition. Everyone has the same 24 hours. The difference between those who experience success and those who spin their wheels is that successful people can actually state their goals and they find different ways to accomplish them. Can you state your goals, or is it easier for you to say what you do not want?

Chews #4 :

Boost Your Creativity:

Create a list of your desires and the steps you need to take to get the result you want.

____

____

____

____

____

____

____

____

____

____

What is stopping your progress? Can you eliminate or modify it?

____

____

____

____

____

____

____

____

____

____

____

Don't forget to schedule time to sleep.

Relationships, Self Care, and Spirituality

These three areas are discussed together because they are all relational, whether the relationship is with self, others, or our spiritual deity. Many of my setbacks over the last 30 years have largely been due to either a failure to put my feelings ahead of others, or a failure to focus on my needs or even to recognize what those needs are. At first this sounded silly and selfish for me to accept about myself. Some of us are nurturers by nature, and some are this way by circumstance. Whatever the case, how do you begin to choose you? Start with what you allow into your body in each setting where you spend your time. Do the people you surround yourself with add positive meaning to your life, or do they require attention that drains you of energy and effort that could be beneficial to you or those you care about? A reevaluation of the relationship, whether it is work-related, personal, or elsewhere needs a closer look from you including a list of "positives" and "negatives" of keeping that relationship. After much self-reflection and honesty about some of my relation-ships with others, myself, and God, I have become much more confident in my abilities to set aside time for my-self. There are various exercises that we can do to im-prove in these three areas to find out what is producing a weakness in our relational foundations. It then becomes easier to say no to others and yes to ourselves.

Why is this so hard for so many of us nurturers? We often work to provide for the needs of others while neglecting our own, which may lead to health issues such as the chronic diseases discussed above which may become advanced before detection. This is why it's so important to set aside uninterrupted time specifically for ourselves. Uninterrupted time alone with God helped me more than any other practice in this book and taught me that it was both physical and emotional hunger that I needed to recognize and nurture. As I began to show more gratitude for everything that I had accomplished, I began to focus more clearly on how to hold on to and appreciate what I had in order to gain more. Not everyone desires to recognize their spirituality in their healing, but I realize that I would not be able to be as healthy without my relationship with God. It's not nearly perfect, but it is mine.

I talk to many clients and potential clients that just don't think they can commit to spending enough time with their families let alone adding the chore of making time for themselves. Alone time for many of us is just unheard of and even evokes guilt in our mommy minds.

How does our handling, or not handling, these various issues translate to the onlooking child that we are molding? I know the last thing we want to do is to make our children feel the anxiety that we feel without a proper explanation for what it is they see in us. Many of us find ourselves getting lost in the list of to do's and may start off with the intent to complete tasks but find ourselves burning out somewhere in the middle. This may manifest in some of the following ways:

- Often showing up late to events, sometimes intentionally because we procrastinate until the very last minute.

- Not showing up at all because we started getting ready at the last minute while anticipating some hindrances might come up, but we were willing to chance it.

- Planning to do things like cook for dinner but ending up telling everyone to eat cereal or order pizza or delivery.

- Consistently getting less than the recommended seven to nine hours of sleep each night.

Chews #5:

**Set Aside 15 Uninterrupted Minutes Two Days
a Week to Do Something for Yourself:**

When was the last time you got your nails or hair done?

____

____

When was the last time you meditated or did something you enjoyed doing?

____

____

When was the last time you said "no" when you really didn't want to do something?

____

____

If you are spiritual, when was the last time you spent time being grounded in your beliefs?

____

____

Happiness

Happiness is defined as a state of well-being and contentment, or joy. Many of us spend an entire life chasing after the one thing that they think will make them consistently happy or bring them joy. I spent almost thirty years chasing after outer sources and accomplishments to bring happiness and joy to my life, when the true source of my joy was always inside of me. It was all about my feeling appreciation for where God allowed me to be and showing unconditional gratitude as I lived each day. Many of us feel we would be happy if we just knew our purpose and focus so heavily on what others are getting done. There is enough success to go around, and another person's wins don't prevent us from having our own successes. Happiness decreases stress and inflammation through raising endorphins, or hormones made by our bodies that relieve pain. How different would your life be if you were to identify a source for your happiness and become focused towards establishing this state of well-being?

Meditation - Studies show that regular meditation for as little as a few minutes a day has health benefits in various areas such as decreasing anxiety, improving sleep, boosting creativity, helping us to deal with stress in general, and even showing improvement in the symptoms of chronic diseases. Meditation doesn't have to be lengthy.

I will introduce a short meditation in the following sentences: Set aside five minutes in your day in a quiet spot. With your feet pressed evenly to the floor, close your eyes, feel the beating of your heart as you slowly inhale, and then exhale to the count of five. Imagine you are in a peaceful, calm place. Repeat this process five times. Open your eyes and remember how it felt to be in that safe serene place as you complete your meditation.

Social media - Social media can be a great business and networking tool but can also be a source of tremendous stress. Various consequences may occur for those who don't use social media responsibly such as sleep loss, anxiety, loss of time and self-care, loss of productivity, and even eye strain. If this could be the case in your life, you can begin to relieve some of the pressures of social media by doing the following: Don't check your social media more than twice a day. Each check should be about the same time of day. Limit the notifications you can see to those that are necessary for your improved productivity, especially if the notifications from a certain source tend to be negative. Choose to follow people and accounts that add positivity and global knowledge to your life. Don't check your social media more than twice a day, each one about the same time of day. Choose to follow people and accounts that add positivity and global knowledge to your life.

As working moms who strive to provide the best for our families, we must monitor a critical part of our mental health—our mindset. Who doesn't want to be around positive, motivated, and ambitious people? The first teachers that all of our children have are us. If we have trouble maintaining a positive mindset, one of the best ways to develop one is with affirmations. It is usually much easier to accomplish something once we know more details about the pathway to achieving the goal. Likewise, planning a healthy lifestyle beginning with meals and food will become much easier once we have a systematic approach for implementing the different food groups into our diets. Along with a newfound level of confidence comes an intuition that we can use to guide us into making these lifestyle choices.

Some of you probably knew much of this information about foods and how to choose them to create your desired effect before reading this guide, but you might have just wanted positive reinforcement that you were moving in the right direction. Many times, we just have to develop our system with our intended results in mind and monitor our situations for results. If there is any negative self-talk holding you back, it's a good idea to recognize that and get to the reason why. Is there something or someone from the past that convinced you that you couldn't make good decisions about your family's well-being? Hopefully that's not the case, but there are ways to reverse such beliefs. I have admitted previously in this guide that I was so unorganized in what I consumed in my diet that I was almost helpless, even with a grocery list, when faced with changes that needed to be made to promote healing. If your wheel showed imbalance in any of the nine areas, you may be experiencing problems with your own mindset.

When I decided to explore ways to improve both mine and my children's health, I was often intimidated by the vast amounts of information on healthy eating and foods to beware of that could be causing more harm than good. I remember feeling at one point like the only thing safe to eat was from a nearby garden or greenhouse and that I was exposing us to cancer or inflammation-causing substances if I went down the wrong aisle of the grocery store. One day a health expert would say that certain vegetables were bad because they contained natural poisonous substances, and the next day I would be wondering if it was not a good idea to feed the kids the tomatoes or the cheese that was in the meal they would eat later. Sometimes too much information is harmful because we tend to overthink and overreact. If this is also you, my advice is to slow down and keep your endpoint of a healthy mind and body for you and your children in mind. Release negative self-talk (in general and about food) and live your life. All of us have made a commitment to be the stewards of this lifestyle to promote healthy outcomes for our loved ones. Let's discuss a few exercises to build that confidence so that we can take charge of our health!

Chews #6:

Show Gratitude Daily for Something, Regardless of Any Obstacles You May Face:

Create positive affirmations that will motivate you for the next five days. Either place them in a bowl to pull out to read daily or write them down to see and repeat daily. Some people even record them to listen to them later.

____

____

____

____

____

One of my favorite affirmations is: No success is too small to celebrate, and I know the small wins prepare me for greater.

Another one of my favorite affirmations is: I am not defined by my mistakes.

Showing gratitude: List three things that you are grateful for and express them before falling asleep at night.

1. ____

2. ____

3. ____

Do each of these for 21 days and reflect on any changes that you have noticed in your life.

Regardless of where you are in your journey to achieving a healthier lifestyle for yourself and those you love, remember that you made the initial steps and even took an assessment to see how balanced you are in your wheel of wellness. That is huge! Take it one day at a time. And, forgive yourself for not being perfect because the one thing we all are is human.

I have always included health and strength as part of success in life. I didn't want to just live. I wanted to feel great. I wanted to be the seventy-year-old out jogging or powerlifting with the forty-year-olds, so I had to start somewhere. I got my first coach and started on my way. Then, I picked up a health coaching certification after a year-long program and started teaching others (along with myself) about the healing powers of foods. I learned about all sorts of healthy greens and plant-based proteins, and I picked up tips for foods that give you energy. For several months, I was almost a Whole Foods groupie.

It has taken me over twenty years to get a good team that includes osteopathic doctors, naturopathic doctors, and a health coach to give me what I need to thrive at this point. At forty years old with twin boys and a newborn daughter, I feel more energetic than I have in a long time. A knowledge of various health conditions as well as the foods and other natural remedies that can be used to prevent or manage them has become very important to me as I have grown into an adult and have become responsible in part for the health of my children.

Physical Activity (Exercise)

Physical activity is very important to supplement eating habits and other lifestyle choices that reduce stress and inflammation. An appropriate amount of exercise is 150 minutes of about 30 minutes, five times a week, with longer durations for weight loss. Appropriate exercise also helps to maximize our basal metabolic rate. It's important to remember that a person's metabolic rate plays a huge role in the amount of calories needed. A couple of different calculations using sex, height, and weight determines just how many calories are needed based on the level of physical activity. It wouldn't be unusual for a sedentary person with all other factors being equal to need 1,000 calories less than a high performing athlete. Reflecting on the concept of bio-individuality, everyone is different. More or less calories may work for some of us.

Optimal weight control can often be maintained if we don't starve ourselves when needing to lose weight because doing so causes the body to go into conservation mode, which ultimately leads to muscle wasting, lowers the metabolic rate, and creates difficulty losing weight. It is a great idea to nourish our bodies with low-calorie whole food snacks that contain carbohydrates and proteins both pre-workout and post-workout, with more protein in the post-workout snacks.

Here are a few tips for healthy exercise habits: combine strength and alignment exercises, manage inflammation through diet and outer foods, listen to cues from your body, and give yourself at least one day a week to recover. Everyone has different stimuli to motivate them. What worked best for me was using my watch to track my physical activity. Whether you're motivated by a certain physical appearance, a workout partner or coach, or even getting a buzz from a watch for not meeting a daily goal, let's get moving!

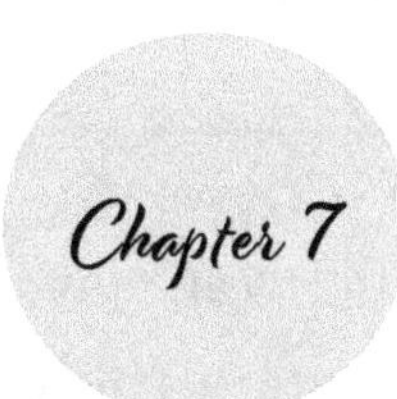

SETTING GOALS AND PLANNING

Look over your self-assessment prior to reviewing the various sections about inner and outer foods. If your wheel isn't rounded, you see where you could use some improvement. A lifestyle that incorporates more plant-based proteins, promotes awareness of your numbers and risk factors, and decreases stressors throughout the various areas on the wheel of wellness is one that tremendously improves the likelihood that you will have fewer symptoms of chronic disease. I envisioned a life at seventy years old where I was free of hypertension, diabetes, sarcoidosis, and had weight issues as the least of my concerns. I also see a similar state of health for my children despite the family history risk factors that we all face. What do you envision for your family, and are you willing to take a few steps toward achieving this?

Chews #7:
Reflect on How Much You Have Progressed Since Completing This Guide:

Which areas in your life needed improvement because they were so much lower on your Wheel of Wellness than the other outer foods?

Wheel of Wellness

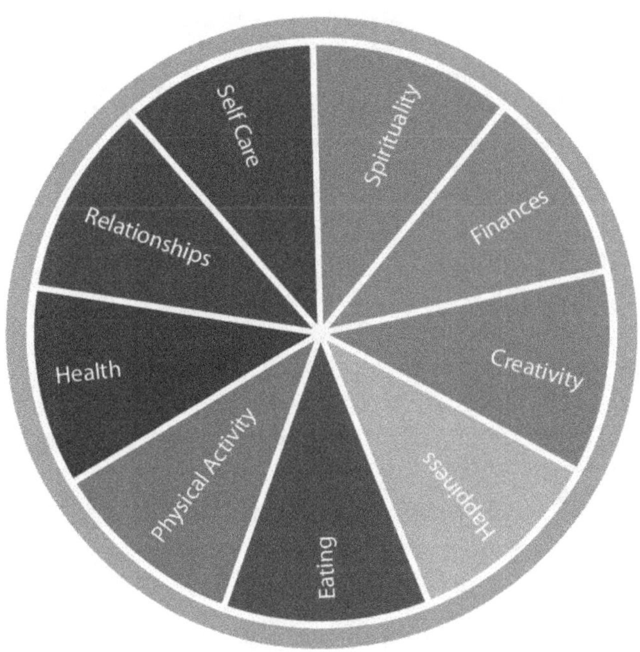

If you are not where you need to be, devise a plan to pull out that outer food and move toward a more balanced circle on your wheel of wellness.

ABOUT THE AUTHOR

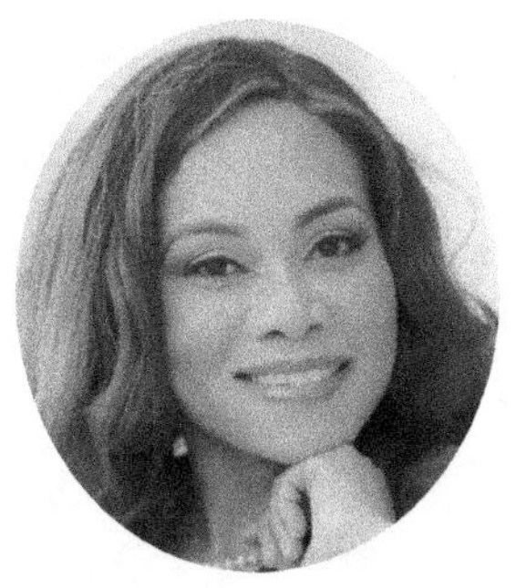

Dr. LaFarra Young-Gaylor is a board-certified pathologist, certified health coach, and co-owner of a Cajun restaurant. After becoming the first African American female pathologist chief resident and pediatric pathologist in her home state of Mississippi and practicing in academic medicine, she entered into private practice. Dr. LaFarra has since performed several hundred pediatric and adult autopsies and has served as a legal consultant for various medicolegal cases in her field. Her mission is to provide working moms with convenient, sustainable, and flavorful products that encourage a healthy lifestyle through coaching, cooking demonstrations, and speaking.

Dr. LaFarra earned her bachelor's degree from Tougaloo College, her medical degree from Boston University School of Medicine, and she is a health coach graduate of the Institute of Integrative Nutrition. Dr. LaFarra is also a contributing author in *The Making of a Medical Mogul, Volumes 2 and 3.*

Dr. LaFarra resides in Jackson, Mississippi, with her three children: Benjamin, Joshua, and Alorya.

Learn more at drlafarra@drlafarramd.com

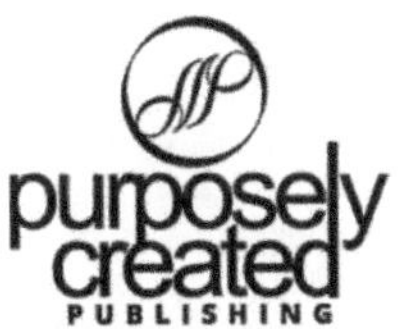

CREATING DISTINCTIVE BOOKS
WITH INTENTIONAL RESULTS

We're a collaborative group of creative masterminds with a mission to produce high-quality books to position you for monumental success in the marketplace.

Our professional team of writers, editors, designers, and marketing strategists work closely together to ensure that every detail of your book is a clear representation of the message in your writing.

Want to know more?
Write to us at info@publishyourgift.com
or call (888) 949-6228

Discover great books, exclusive offers, and more at
www.PublishYourGift.com

Connect with us on social media

@publishyourgift

www.ingramcontent.com/pod-product-compliance
Lightning Source LLC
Chambersburg PA
CBHW061538050726

47593CB00002B/819